LOW FAT AIR FRYER
FRYER

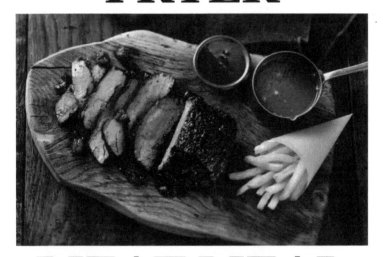

MEAT MEAL
PREP

Celine Montero

Welcome!

"Low Fat Air Fryer Meal Prep" is a series I created to walk you through delicious recipes selected by myself. As you may already know, the air fryer is a fantastic tool anybody can use to quickly prepare our meals, through a healthy cooking method.

The fact is that's the latest hottest kitchen appliance .

BENEFITS OF THE AIR FRYER

- *Less Cooking Time*

It cooks your food using the fan to circulate the hot air on all parts of your food. Thanks to the design, it cooks faster than a regular oven. You are able to cook your meal in 15mins, while it takes much more to do in in an oven.

• *Energy Efficient*

When there's a heatwave you will have the air fryer cook without influencing your home temperature. most people prefer to work with gadgets that show to be environmentally friendly - This is one such gadget. Hence most people prefer the air fryer rather than a regular oven.

• *Super Easy To Clean*

For those people with problems of cleaning, do not worry at all because you won't have to spend much time cleaning with this gadget.

You can place the parts directly in your dishwasher.

• *Super Easy To Use*

Most of the air fryers have only 2 buttons to control the entire appliance. The only two things you need to do are setting the temperature and time, then let the food cook after you shaked it a few times.

• *It Is Versatile*

With just the air fryer, you can deep fry the food, stir fry, reheat, broil, bake or roast it. You cannot have in your kitchen tools able do only one thing or cook just one kind of food.

The recipes this series of books contains are selected and divided by categories in 8 cookbooks, to made you enjoy as best this (in my opinion) revolutionary way to cook foods. I hope you will enjoy and find all these recipes interesting and helpful to set up your daily meal plan.

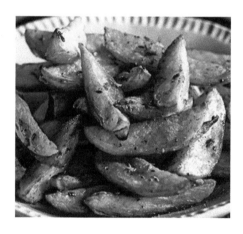

Celine Montero

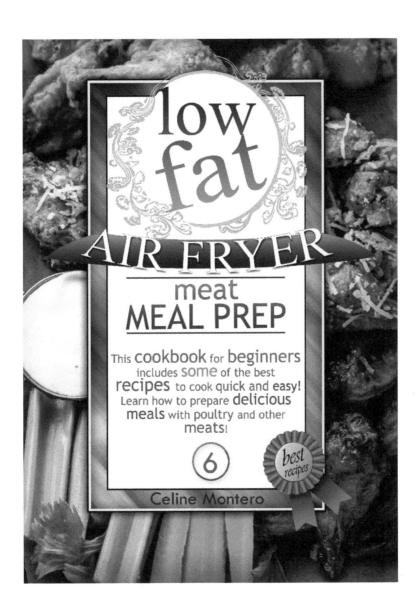

low fat

AIR FRYER

meat
MEAL PREP

This **cookbook** for **beginners**
includes **some** of the best
recipes to cook **quick** and **easy!**
Learn how to prepare **delicious**
meals with poultry and other
meats!

6

best recipes

Celine Montero

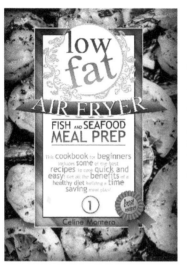

LOW FAT AIR FRYER
FISH AND SEAFOOD MEAL PREP

This cookbook for beginners includes some of the best recipes to cook quick and easy! Get all the benefits of a healthy diet building a time saving meal plan!

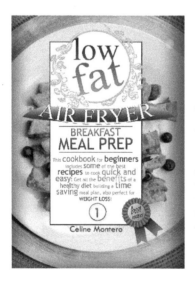

LOW FAT AIR FRYER
BREAKFAST MEAL PREP

This cookbook for beginners includes some of the best recipes to cook quick and easy! Get all the benefits of a healthy diet building a time saving meal plan, also perfect for weight loss!

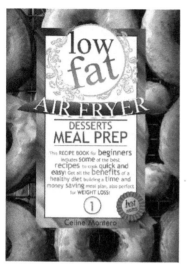

LOW FAT AIR FRYER
DESSERTS MEAL PREP

This recipe book for beginners includes some of the best recipes to cook quick and easy! Get all the benefits of a healthy diet building a time and money saving meal plan, also perfect for weight loss!

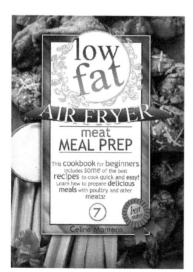

LOW FAT AIR FRYER
MEAT MEAL PREP

This cookbook for beginners includes some of the best recipes to cook quick and easy! Learn how to prepare delicious meals with poultry and other meats!

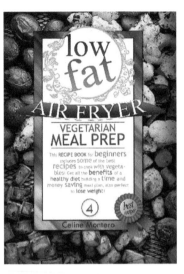

LOW FAT AIR FRYER
VEGETARIAN MEAL PREP

This recipe book for beginners includes some of the best recipes to cook with vegetables! Get all the benefits of a healthy diet building a time and money saving meal plan, also perfect to lose weight!

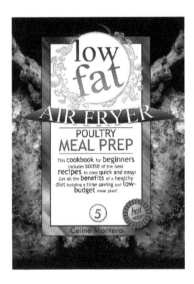

LOW FAT AIR FRYER
POULTRY MEAL PREP

This cookbook for beginners includes some of the best recipes to cook quick and easy! Get all the benefits of a healthy diet building a time saving and low-budget meal plan!

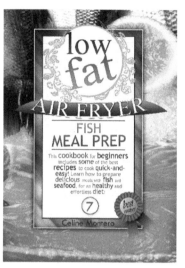

LOW FAT AIR FRYER
POULTRY MEAL PREP

This cookbook for beginners includes some of the best recipes to cook quick-and-easy! Learn how to prepare delicious meals with fish and seafood,
for a healthy and effortless diet!

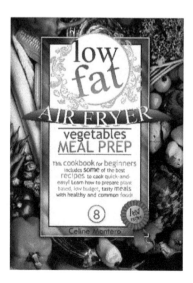

LOW FAT AIR FRYER
VEGETABLES MEAL PREP

This cookbook for beginners includes some of the best recipes to cook quick-and-easy! Learn how to prepare plant-based, low-budget and tasty meals, with healthy and common food, ideal for weight loss!

11

PLANT-BASED DIET WITH AIR FRYER

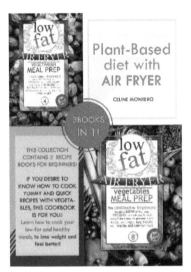

This collection contains 2 recipe books for beginners! If you desire to know how to cook yummy and quick recipes with vegetables, this cookbook is for you! Learn how to cook your low-fat and healthy meals, to lose weight and feel better!

THE BEST AIR FRYER COOKBOOK

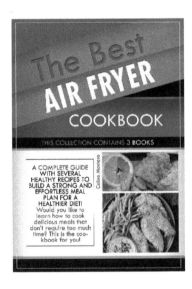

THIS COLLECTION CONTAINS 3 BOOKS: a complete guide with several healthy recipes to build a strong and effortless meal plan for a healthier diet! Would you like to learn how to cook delicious meals that don't require too much time? This is the cookbook for you!

Table of Contents

MEAT

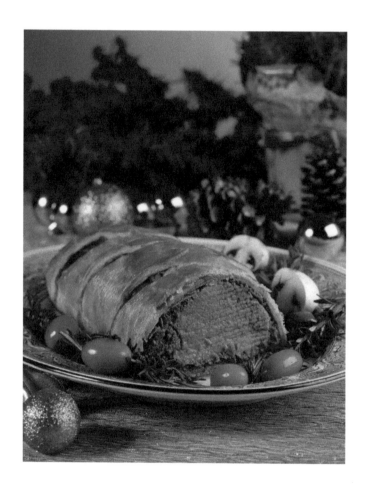

Simple & Juicy Steak

Preparation Time: 10 minutes Cooking Time: 13 minutes Serve: 2

Ingredients:

- 12 oz ribeye steak
- 1 tsp steak seasoning
- 1 tbsp olive oil
- Pepper Salt

Directions:

Coat steak with oil and season with steak seasoning, pepper, and salt. Place the cooking tray in the air fryer basket. Select Air Fry mode. Set time to 13 minutes and temperature 400 F then press START. The air fryer display will prompt you to ADD FOOD once the temperature is reached then place steak in the air fryer basket. Serve and enjoy.

Pork Chop Fries

Preparation Time: 10 minutes Cooking Time: 15 minutes Serve: 4

Ingredients:

- 1 lb pork chops, cut into fries
- 1/2 cup parmesan cheese, grated
- 3.5 oz pork rinds, crushed
- 1/2 cup ranch dressing
- Pepper Salt

Directions:

In a shallow dish, mix together crushed pork rinds, parmesan cheese, pepper, and salt. Add pork chop pieces and ranch dressing into the zip-lock bag, seal bag, and shake well. Remove pork chop pieces from zip-lock bag and coat with crushed pork rind mixture. Place the cooking tray in the air fryer basket. Line air fryer basket with parchment paper. Select Bake mode. Set time to 15 minutes and temperature 400 F then press START. The air fryer display will prompt you to ADD FOOD once the temperature is reached then place breaded pork chop fries in the air fryer basket. Serve and enjoy.

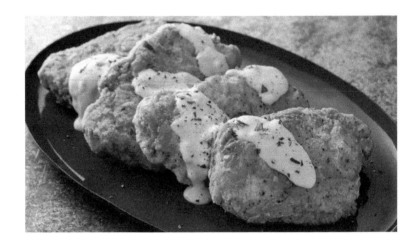

Spicy Pork Patties

Preparation Time: 10 minutes Cooking Time: 10 minutes Serve: 2

Ingredients:

- 1/2 lb ground pork
- 1 tbsp Cajun seasoning
- 1 egg, lightly beaten
- 1/2 cup almond flour
- Pepper Salt

Directions:

Add all ingredients into the large bowl and mix until well combined. Make two equal shapes of patties from the meat mixture. Select Air Fry mode. Set time to 10 minutes and temperature 360 F then press START. The air fryer display will prompt you to ADD FOOD once the temperature is reached then place patties in the air fryer basket. Serve and enjoy.

Spicy Parmesan Pork Chops

Preparation Time: 10 minutes Cooking Time: 9 minutes Serve: 2

Ingredients:

- 2 pork chops, boneless
- 1 tsp paprika
- 3 tbsp parmesan cheese, grated
- 1/3 cup almond flour
- 1 tsp Cajun seasoning
- 1 tsp dried mixed herbs

Directions:

In a shallow bowl, mix together parmesan cheese, almond flour, paprika, mixed herbs, and Cajun seasoning. Spray pork chops with cooking spray and coat with parmesan cheese. Select Air Fry mode. Set time to 9 minutes and temperature 350 F then press START. The air fryer display will prompt you to ADD FOOD once the temperature is reached then place breaded pork chops in the air fryer basket. Turn pork chops halfway through. Serve and enjoy.

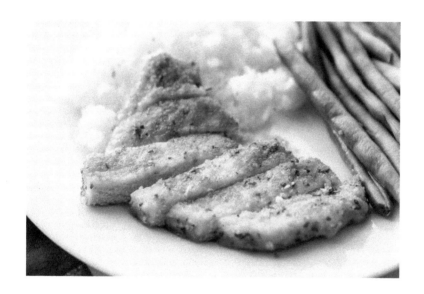

Air Fried Pork Bites

Preparation Time: 10 minutes Cooking Time: 15 minutes Serve: 4

Ingredients:

- 1 lb pork belly, cut into 1-inch cubes
- 1 tsp soy sauce
- Pepper Salt

Directions:

In a bowl, toss pork cubes with soy sauce, pepper, and salt. Select Air Fry mode. Set time to 15 minutes and temperature 400 F then press START. The air fryer display will prompt you to ADD FOOD once the temperature is reached then place pork cubes in the air fryer basket. Serve and enjoy.

Steak Tips

Preparation Time: 10 minutes Cooking Time: 5 minutes Serve: 3

Ingredients:

- 1 lb steak, cut into cubes
- 1 tsp olive oil
- 1 tsp Montreal steak seasoning
- Pepper Salt

Directions:

In a bowl, add steak cubes and remaining ingredients and toss well. Select Air Fry mode. Set time to 5 minutes and temperature 400 F then press START. The air fryer display will prompt you to ADD FOOD once the temperature is reached then place steak cubes in the air fryer basket. Serve and enjoy.

Ranch Patties

Preparation Time: 10 minutes Cooking Time: 12 minutes Serve: 4

Ingredients:

- 1 lb ground beef
- 1/2 tsp dried dill
- 1/2 tsp onion powder
- 1/2 tsp garlic powder
- 2 tsp dried parsley
- 1/8 tsp dried dill
- 1/2 tsp paprika
- Pepper Salt

Directions:

Add all ingredients into the large bowl and mix until well combined. Make 4 even shape patties from meat mixture. Select Air Fry mode. Set time to 12 minutes and temperature 350 F then press START. The air fryer display will prompt you to ADD FOOD once the temperature is reached then place patties in the air fryer basket. Serve and enjoy.

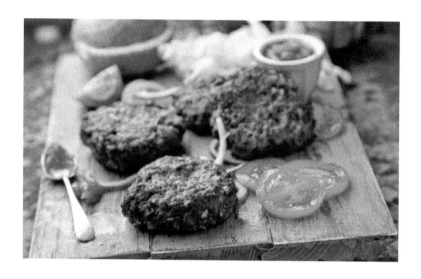

Easy Beef Kebabs

Preparation Time: 10 minutes Cooking Time: 10 minutes Serve: 4

Ingredients:

- 1 lb beef chuck ribs, cut into
- 1-inch pieces
- 1/2 onion, cut into 1-inch pieces
- 2 tbsp soy sauce
- 1/3 cup sour cream
- 1 bell pepper, cut into
- 1-inch pieces

Directions:

Add meat pieces, soy sauce, and sour cream into the mixing bowl and mix well. Cover bowl and place in the refrigerator overnight. Thread marinated meat, onion, and bell peppers pieces onto the soaked wooden skewers. Select Air Fry mode. Set time to 10 minutes and temperature 400 F then press START. The air fryer display will prompt you to ADD FOOD once the temperature is reached then place skewers in the air fryer basket. Turn halfway through. Serve and enjoy.

Air Fryer Beef Fajitas

Preparation Time: 10 minutes Cooking Time: 8 minutes Serve: 4

Ingredients:

- 1 lb steak, sliced
- 1/2 tbsp chili powder
- 3 tbsp olive oil
- 2 bell peppers, sliced
- 1 tsp garlic powder
- 1 tsp paprika
- 1 tsp cumin
- Pepper Salt

Directions:

In a mixing bowl, toss sliced steak with remaining ingredients. Select Air Fry mode. Set time to 8 minutes and temperature 390 F then press START. The air fryer display will prompt you to ADD FOOD once the temperature is reached then place fajitas in the air fryer basket. Serve and enjoy.

Juicy Pork Tenderloin

Preparation Time: 10 minutes Cooking Time: 20 minutes Serve: 4

Ingredients:

- 1 1/2 lbs pork tenderloin
- 2 tbsp olive oil
- 1 tsp garlic powder
- 1 tsp Italian seasoning
- 1/4 tsp pepper
- 1 tsp sea salt

Directions:

Rub pork tenderloin with 1 tablespoon of olive oil. Mix together garlic powder, Italian seasoning, pepper, and salt and rub over pork tenderloin. Heat remaining oil in a pan over medium-high heat. Add pork tenderloin in hot oil and cook until brown Select Bake mode. Set time to 15 minutes and temperature 400 F then press START. The air fryer display will prompt you to ADD FOOD once the temperature is reached then place pork tenderloin in the air fryer basket. Serve and enjoy.

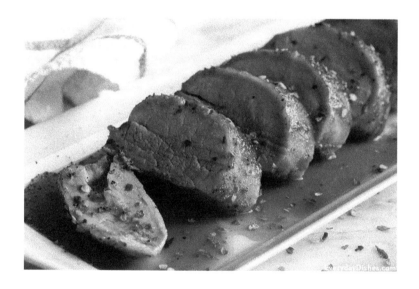

Lemon Pepper Pork

Preparation Time: 10 minutes Cooking Time: 15 minutes Serve: 4

Ingredients:

- 4 pork chops, boneless
- 1 tsp lemon
- pepper seasoning Salt

Directions:

Season pork chops with lemon pepper seasoning, and salt. Select Air Fry mode. Set time to 15 minutes and temperature 400 F then press START. The air fryer display will prompt you to ADD FOOD once the temperature is reached then place pork chops in the air fryer basket. Serve and enjoy.

Stuffed Pork Chops

Preparation Time: 10 minutes Cooking Time: 35 minutes Serve: 4

Ingredients:

- 4 pork chops, boneless and thick-cut
- 2 tbsp olives, chopped
- 2 tbsp sun-dried tomatoes, chopped
- 1/2 cup feta cheese, crumbled
- 2 garlic cloves, minced
- 2 tbsp fresh parsley, chopped

Directions:

In a bowl, combine together feta cheese, garlic, parsley, olives, and sun-dried tomatoes. Stuff cheese mixture all the pork chops. Season pork chops with pepper and salt. Select Bake mode. Set time to 35 minutes and temperature 375 F then press START. The air fryer display will prompt you to ADD FOOD once the temperature is reached then place stuffed pork chops in the air fryer basket. Serve and enjoy

Air Fryer Lamb Chops

Preparation Time: 10 minutes Cooking Time: 12 minutes Serve: 4

Ingredients:

- 4 lamb chops
- 2 garlic clove, minced
- 3 tbsp olive oil
- Pepper Salt

Directions:

In a small bowl, mix together thyme and oil. Season lamb chops with pepper and salt and rubs with thyme mixture. Select Air Fry mode. Set time to 12 minutes and temperature 400 F then press START. The air fryer display will prompt you to ADD FOOD once the temperature is reached then place lamb chops in the air fryer basket. Turn halfway through. Serve and enjoy.

Breaded Pork Chops

Preparation Time: 10 minutes Cooking Time: 20 minutes Serve: 4

Ingredients:

- 4 pork chops, boneless
- 1/4 cup parmesan cheese, grated
- 1 cup almond meal
- 1/2 tbsp black pepper
- 1 tbsp onion powder
- 1 tbsp garlic powder
- 2 eggs, lightly beaten
- 1/2 tsp sea salt

Directions:

In a bowl, mix together almond meal, parmesan cheese, onion powder, garlic powder, pepper, and salt. Whisk eggs in a shallow dish. Dip pork chops into the egg then coat with almond meal mixture. Select Air Fry mode. Set time to 20 minutes and temperature 350 F then press

START. The air fryer display will prompt you to ADD FOOD once the temperature is reached then place breaded pork chops in the air fryer basket. Turn pork chops halfway through. Serve and enjoy.

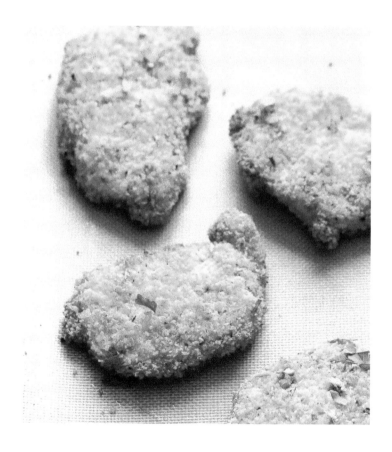

Creole Seasoned Pork Chops

Preparation Time: 10 minutes Cooking Time: 12 minutes Serve: 6

Ingredients:

- 1 1/2 lbs pork chops, boneless
- 1/4 cup parmesan cheese, grated
- 1/3 cup almond flour
- 1 tsp paprika
- 1 tsp Creole seasoning
- 1 tsp garlic powder

Directions:

Add all ingredients except pork chops into the zip-lock bag. Add pork chops into the bag. Seal bag and shake well. Remove pork chops from the zip-lock bag. Select Air Fry mode. Set time to 12 minutes and temperature 360 F then press START. The air fryer display will prompt you to ADD FOOD once the temperature is reached then place pork chops in the air fryer basket. Serve and enjoy.

Coconut Pork Chops

Preparation Time: 10 minutes Cooking Time: 14 minutes Serve: 4

Ingredients:

- 4 pork chops
- 1 tbsp coconut oil
- 1 tbsp coconut butter
- 2 tsp parsley
- 2 tsp garlic, grated
- Pepper Salt

Directions:

In a large bowl, mix together with seasonings, garlic, butter, and coconut oil. Add pork chops to the bowl and mix well. Place in refrigerator overnight. Select Air Fry mode. Set time to 14 minutes and temperature 350 F then press START. The air fryer display will prompt you to ADD FOOD once the temperature is reached then place marinated pork chops in the air fryer basket. Turn pork chops halfway through. Serve and enjoy.

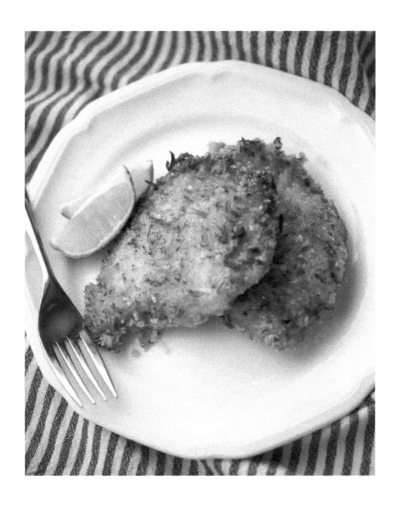

Jerk Pork Cubes

Preparation Time: 10 minutes Cooking Time: 20 minutes Serve: 4

Ingredients:

- 1
- 1/2 lbs pork butt, cut into pieces
- 1/4 cup jerk paste
- Pepper Salt

Directions:

Add meat and jerk paste into the bowl and mix well and place in refrigerator overnight. Select Air Fry mode. Set time to 20 minutes and temperature 390 F then press START. The air fryer display will prompt you to ADD FOOD once the temperature is reached then place marinated pork pieces in the air fryer basket. Stir halfway through. Serve and enjoy.

Smokey Steaks

Preparation Time: 10 minutes Cooking Time: 7 minutes Serve: 2

Ingredients:

- 12 oz steaks
- 1 tbsp Montreal steak seasoning
- 1 tsp liquid smoke
- 1 tbsp soy sauce
- 1/2 tbsp cocoa powder
- Pepper Salt

Directions:

Add steak, liquid smoke, soy sauce, and steak seasonings into the large zip-lock bag. Shake well and place it in the refrigerator overnight. Select Air Fry mode. Set time to 7 minutes and temperature 375 F then press START. The air fryer display will prompt you to ADD FOOD once the temperature is reached then place steaks in the air fryer basket. Turn steaks after 5 minutes. Serve and enjoy.

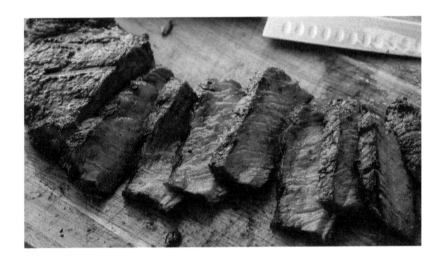

Simple Beef Kabab

Preparation Time: 10 minutes Cooking Time: 10 minutes Serve: 4

Ingredients:

- 1 lb ground beef
- 2 tbsp kabab spice mix
- 1 tbsp garlic, minced
- 1 tbsp olive oil
- 1 tsp salt

Directions:

Add all ingredients into the mixing bowl and mix until well combined. Place in refrigerator for 30 minutes. Divide mixture into the 4 equal portions and make sausage shape kabab. Select Air Fry mode. Set time to 10 minutes and temperature 370 F then press START. The air fryer display will prompt you to ADD FOOD once the temperature is reached then place kabab in the air fryer basket. Serve and enjoy.

Spicy Pork Tenderloin

Preparation Time: 10 minutes Cooking Time: 35 minutes Serve: 6

Ingredients:

- 2 pork tenderloin

For rub:

- 1 tbsp smoked paprika
- 1 tbsp garlic powder
- 1 tbsp onion powder
- 1/2 tbsp salt

Directions:

In a small bowl, combine together all rub ingredients. Coat pork tenderloin with the rub. Heat ovenproof pan over medium-high heat. Spray pan with cooking spray. Sear pork on all sides until lightly golden brown. Select Bake mode. Set time to 30 minutes and temperature 400 F then press START. The air fryer display will prompt you to ADD FOOD once the temperature is reached then place pork tenderloin in the air fryer basket. Serve and enjoy.

Garlic Thyme Lamb Chops

Preparation Time: 5 minutes Cooking Time: 12 minutes Serve: 4

Ingredients:

- 4 lamb chops
- 4 garlic clove, minced
- 3 tbsp olive oil
- Pepper Salt

Directions:

In a small bowl, mix together oil and garlic. Season lamb chops with pepper and salt and rubs with oil and garlic mixture. Select Bake mode. Set time to 12 minutes and temperature 400 F then press START. The air fryer display will prompt you to ADD FOOD once the temperature is reached then place lamb chops in the air fryer basket. Turn lamb chops halfway through. Serve and enjoy.

Delicious Herb Beef Patties

Preparation Time: 10 minutes Cooking Time: 45 minutes Serve: 4

Ingredients:

- 10 oz beef minced
- 1/4 tsp ginger paste
- 1 1/2 tsp mixed herbs
- 1 tsp basil
- 1 tsp tomato puree
- 1 tsp garlic puree
- 1/2 tsp mustard
- Pepper Salt

Directions:

Add all ingredients into the large bowl and mix until well combined. Make patties from meat mixture. Select Air

Fry mode. Set time to 45 minutes and temperature 375 F then press START. The air fryer display will prompt you to ADD FOOD once the temperature is reached then place patties in the air fryer basket. Serve and enjoy.

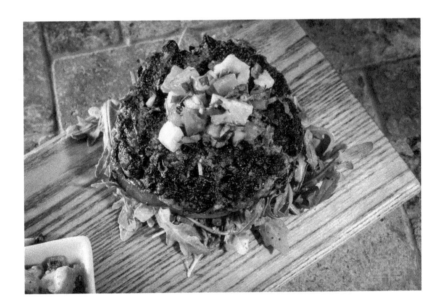

Roasted Sirloin Steak

Preparation Time: 10 minutes Cooking Time: 30 minutes Serve: 6

Ingredients:

- 2 lbs sirloin steak, cut into
- 1-inch cubes
- 2 garlic cloves, minced
- 3 tbsp fresh lemon juice
- 1 tsp dried oregano
- 1/4 tsp thyme
- 1/4 cup water
- 1/4 cup olive oil
- 2 cups fresh parsley, chopped
- 1/2 tsp pepper
- 1 tsp salt

Directions:

Add all ingredients except beef into the large bowl and mix well. Pour bowl mixture into the large zip-lock bag. Add steak cubes into the bag and seal bag and place in refrigerator for 1 hour. Place marinated beef on a baking dish and cover dish with foil. Select Bake mode. Set time to 30 minutes and temperature 400 F then press START. The air fryer display will prompt you to ADD FOOD once the temperature is reached then place the baking dish in the air fryer basket. Serve and enjoy.

Basil Cheese Lamb Patties

Preparation Time: 10 minutes Cooking Time: 8 minutes Serve: 4

Ingredients:

- 1 lb ground lamb
- 1 cup goat cheese, crumbled
- 1 tbsp garlic, minced
- 6 basil leaves, minced
- 1 tsp chili powder
- 1/4 cup mint leaves, minced
- 1/4 cup fresh parsley, chopped
- 1 tsp dried oregano
- 1/4 tsp pepper
- 1/2 tsp kosher salt

Directions:

Add all ingredients into the mixing bowl and mix until well combined. Make four equal shape patties from the meat mixture. Select Bake mode. Set time to 8 minutes and temperature 400 F then press START. The air fryer display will prompt you to ADD FOOD once the temperature is reached then place patties in the air fryer basket. Turn patties halfway through. Serve and enjoy.

Air Fryer Stew Meat

Preparation Time: 10 minutes Cooking Time: 25 minutes Serve: 4

Ingredients:

- 1 lb beef stew meat, cut into strips
- 1/2 lime juice
- 1 tbsp olive oil
- 1/2 tbsp ground cumin
- 1 tbsp garlic powder
- 1/2 tsp onion powder
- Pepper Salt

Directions:

Add meat and remaining ingredients into the mixing bowl and mix well. Select Air Fry mode. Set time to 25 minutes and temperature 380 F then press START. The air fryer display will prompt you to ADD FOOD once the temperature is reached then place stew meat in the air fryer basket. Stir halfway through Serve and enjoy.

Stuffed Bell Peppers

Preparation Time: 10 minutes Cooking Time: 20 minutes Serve: 2

Ingredients:

- 8 oz ground pork
- 2 bell peppers, remove stems and seeds
- 1/2 cup tomato sauce
- 4 oz mozzarella cheese, shredded
- 1 tsp olive oil
- 1 garlic clove, minced
- 1/2 onion, chopped
- 1/2 tsp pepper
- 1/2 tsp salt

Directions:

Sauté garlic and onion in the olive oil in a small pan until softened. Add meat, 1/4 cup tomato sauce, half cheese, pepper, and salt and stir to combine. Stuff meat mixture into each pepper and top with remaining cheese and tomato sauce. Select Air Fry mode. Set time to 20 minutes and temperature 390 F then press START. The air fryer display will prompt you to ADD FOOD once the temperature is reached then place stuffed pepper in the air fryer basket. Serve and enjoy.

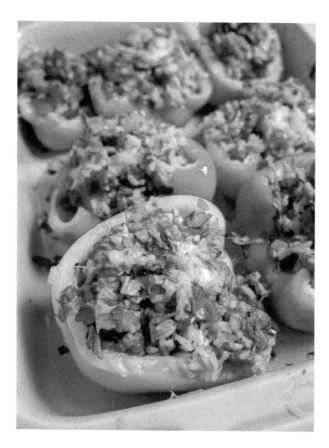

Ranch Pork Chops

Preparation Time: 10 minutes Cooking Time: 35 minutes Serve: 4

Ingredients:

- 4 pork chops, boneless
- 1 oz ranch seasoning
- 1 1/2 tbsp olive oil

Directions:

Brush pork chops with oil and rub with ranch seasoning. Select Air Fry mode. Set time to 35 minutes and temperature 400 F then press START. The air fryer display will prompt you to ADD FOOD once the temperature is reached then place pork chops in the air fryer basket. Serve and enjoy.

Taco Stuffed Peppers

Preparation Time: 10 minutes Cooking Time: 8 minutes Serve: 12

Ingredients:

- 6 jalapeno peppers, cut in half & remove seeds
- 1 1/2 tbsp taco seasoning
- 1/2 lb ground beef
- 1/4 cup goat cheese, crumbled

Directions:

Browned the meat in a large pan. Remove pan from heat. Add taco seasoning to the ground meat and mix well. Stuff meat into each jalapeno half. Select Air Fry mode. Set time to 6 minutes and temperature 320 F then press START. The air fryer display will prompt you to ADD FOOD once the temperature is reached then place jalapeno halves in the air fryer basket. Sprinkle cheese on top of peppers and cook for 2 minutes more. Serve and enjoy.

Breaded Pork Chops

Preparation Time: 10 minutes Cooking Time: 15 minutes Serve: 2

Ingredients:

- 2 pork chops, bone-in
- 1 tbsp olive oil
- 1 cup pork rinds, crushed
- 1/2 tsp paprika
- 1/2 tsp dried parsley
- 1/2 tsp garlic powder
- 1/2 tsp onion powder
- 1/4 tsp chili powder

Directions:

In a large bowl, mix together pork rinds, garlic powder, onion powder, parsley, chili powder, and paprika. Brush pork chops with oil and coat with pork rind mixture. Select Air Fry mode. Set time to 15 minutes and temperature 400 F then press START. The air fryer display will prompt you to ADD FOOD once the temperature is reached then place pork chops in the air fryer basket. Turn pork chops after 10 minutes. Serve and enjoy.

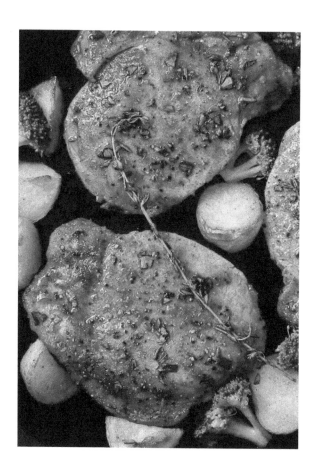

Garlicky Pork Chops

Preparation Time: 10 minutes Cooking Time: 20 minutes Serve: 8

Ingredients:

- 8 pork chops, boneless
- 6 garlic cloves, minced
- 1/4 tsp pepper
- 3/4 cup parmesan cheese
- 2 tbsp butter, melted
- 2 tbsp coconut oil
- 1 tsp thyme
- 1 tbsp parsley
- 1/2 tsp sea salt

Directions:

In a small bowl, mix together butter, garlic, pepper, thyme, parsley, parmesan cheese, coconut oil, and salt. Brush butter mixture on top of pork chops. Select Air Fry mode. Set time to 20 minutes and temperature 400 F then press START. The air fryer display will prompt you to ADD FOOD once the temperature is reached then place pork chops in the air fryer basket. Turn pork chops halfway through. Serve and enjoy.

Dijon Pork Chops

Preparation Time: 10 minutes Cooking Time: 12 minutes Serve: 4

Ingredients:

- 4 pork chops
- 1 tbsp garlic, minced
- 4 tbsp Dijon mustard
- Pepper Salt

Directions:

In a small bowl, mix together mustard, garlic, pepper, and salt Brush pork chops with mustard mixture. Select Air Fry mode. Set time to 12 minutes and temperature 350 F then press START. The air fryer display will prompt you to ADD FOOD once the temperature is reached then place pork chops in the air fryer basket. Turn pork chops halfway through. Serve and enjoy.

Pecan Dijon Pork Chops

Preparation Time: 10 minutes Cooking Time: 12 minutes Serve: 6

Ingredients:

- 1 egg
- 6 pork chops, boneless
- 2 garlic cloves, minced
- 1 tbsp water
- 1 tsp Dijon mustard
- 1 tsp garlic powder
- 1 tsp onion powder
- 2 tsp Italian seasoning
- 1/3 cup arrowroot
- 1 cup pecans, finely chopped
- 1/4 tsp salt

Directions:

In a shallow bowl, whisk the egg with garlic, water, and Dijon mustard. In a separate shallow bowl, mix together arrowroot, pecans, Italian seasoning, onion powder, garlic powder, and salt. Dip pork chop in the egg mixture and coat with arrowroot mixture. Place the cooking tray in the air fryer basket. Select Air Fry mode. Set time to 12 minutes and temperature 400 F then press START. The air fryer display will prompt you to ADD FOOD once the temperature is reached then place coated pork chops in the air fryer basket. Turn pork chops halfway through. Serve and enjoy.

Marinated Ribeye Steaks

Preparation Time: 10 minutes Cooking Time: 12 minutes Serve: 4

Ingredients:

- 2 large ribeye steaks,
- 1 1/2-inch thick
- 1 1/2 tbsp Montreal steak seasoning
- 1/2 cup low-sodium soy sauce
- 1/4 cup olive oil

Directions:

Add soy sauce, oil, and Montreal steak seasoning in a large zip-lock bag. Add steaks in a zip-lock bag. Seal bag shakes well and places in the refrigerator for 2 hours. Place the cooking tray in the air fryer basket. Select Air Fry mode. Set time to 12 minutes and temperature 400 F then press START. The air fryer display will prompt you to ADD FOOD once the temperature is reached then remove steaks from marinade and place in the air fryer basket. Turn steaks halfway through. Serve and enjoy.

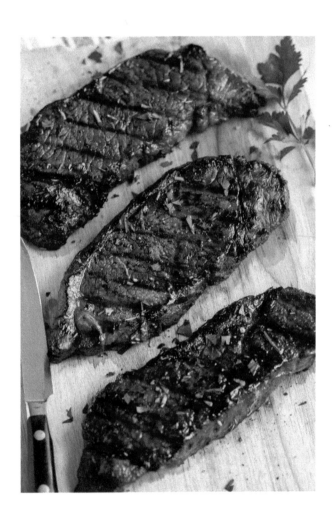

Pork Kebabs

Preparation Time: 10 minutes Cooking Time: 15 minutes Serve: 6

Ingredients:

- 2 lbs country-style pork ribs, cut into cubes
- 1/4 cup soy sauce
- 1/2 cup olive oil
- 1 tbsp Italian seasoning

Directions:

Add soy sauce, oil, Italian seasoning, and pork cubes into the zip-lock bag, seal bag and place in the refrigerator for 4 hours. Remove pork cubes from marinade and place the cubes on wooden skewers. Place the cooking tray in the air fryer basket. Line air fryer basket with parchment paper. Select Bake mode. Set time to 15 minutes and temperature 380 F then press START. The air fryer display will prompt you to ADD FOOD once the temperature is reached then place pork skewers in the air fryer basket. Serve and enjoy

Herb Pork Chops

Preparation Time: 10 minutes Cooking Time: 15 minutes Serve: 4

Ingredients:

- 4 pork chops
- 2 tsp oregano
- 2 tsp thyme
- 2 tsp sage
- 1 tsp garlic powder
- 1 tsp paprika
- 1 tsp rosemary
- Pepper Salt

Directions:

Spray pork chops with cooking spray. Mix together garlic powder, paprika, rosemary, oregano, thyme, sage, pepper, and salt and rub over pork chops. Select Air Fry mode. Set time to 15 minutes and temperature 360 F then press START. The air fryer display will prompt you to ADD FOOD once the temperature is reached then place pork chops in the air fryer basket. Turn pork chops halfway through. Serve and enjoy.

Pork Chops

Preparation Time: 10 minutes Cooking Time: 14 minutes Serve: 2

Ingredients:

- 2 pork chops
- 1 tsp paprika
- 1 tsp garlic powder
- 1 tsp olive oil
- Pepper Salt

Directions:

Brush pork chops with olive oil and season with garlic powder, paprika, pepper, and salt. Select Air Fry mode. Set time to 14 minutes and temperature 360 F then press START. The air fryer display will prompt you to ADD FOOD once the temperature is reached then place pork chops in the air fryer basket. Turn pork chops halfway through.

Rosemary Beef Tips

Preparation Time: 10 minutes Cooking Time: 12 minutes Serve: 4

Ingredients:

- 1 lb steak, cut into 1-inch cubes
- 1 tsp paprika
- 2 tsp onion powder
- 1 tsp garlic powder
- 2 tbsp coconut aminos
- 2 tsp rosemary, crushed
- Pepper Salt

Directions:

Add meat and remaining ingredients into the mixing bowl and mix well and let it sit for 5 minutes. Select Air Fry mode. Set time to 12 minutes and temperature 380 F then press START. The air fryer display will prompt you to ADD FOOD once the temperature is reached then place steak cubes in the air fryer basket. Stir halfway through. Serve and enjoy.

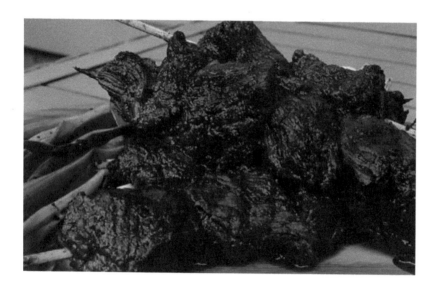

Sirloin Steak

Preparation Time: 10 minutes Cooking Time: 14 minutes Serve: 2

Ingredients:

- 1 lb sirloin steaks
- 1/2 tsp garlic powder
- 1/4 tsp onion powder
- 1 tsp olive oil
- Pepper Salt

Directions:

Brush steak with olive oil and rub with garlic powder, onion powder, pepper, and salt. Select Air Fry mode. Set time to 14 minutes and temperature 400 F then press START. The air fryer display will prompt you to ADD FOOD once the temperature is reached then place steaks in the air fryer basket. Turn steak halfway through. Serve and enjoy.

Steak & Mushrooms

Preparation Time: 10 minutes Cooking Time: 18 minutes Serve: 4

Ingredients:

- 1 lb steaks, cut into 1-inch cubes
- 2 tbsp olive oil
- 8 oz mushrooms, halved
- 1/2 tsp garlic powder
- 1 tsp Worcestershire sauce
- Pepper Salt

Directions:

Add steak cubes and remaining ingredients into the mixing bowl and toss until well coated. Select Air Fry mode. Set time to 18 minutes and temperature 400 F then press START. The air fryer display will prompt you to ADD FOOD once the temperature is reached then place steak and mushrooms in the air fryer basket. Stir halfway through. Serve and enjoy.

Flavorful Burger Patties

Preparation Time: 10 minutes Cooking Time: 15 minutes Serve: 4

Ingredients:

- 1 lb ground lamb
- 1/4 tsp cayenne pepper
- 1/4 cup fresh parsley, chopped
- 1/4 cup onion, minced
- 1 tbsp garlic, minced
- 1/2 tsp ground allspice
- 1 tsp ground cinnamon
- 1 tsp ground coriander
- 1 tsp ground cumin
- 1/4 tsp pepper
- 1 tsp kosher salt

Directions:

Add all ingredients into the large bowl and mix until well combined. Make 4 patties from the meat mixture. Select Bake mode. Set time to 14 minutes and temperature 375 F then press START. The air fryer display will prompt you to ADD FOOD once the temperature is reached then place patties in the air fryer basket. Turn patties halfway through. Serve and enjoy

Baked Beef & Broccoli

Preparation Time: 10 minutes Cooking Time: 25 minutes Serve: 2

Ingredients:

- 1/2 cup broccoli florets
- 1/2 lb beef stew meat, cut into pieces
- 1 onion, sliced
- 1 tbsp vinegar
- 1 tbsp olive oil
- Pepper Salt

Directions:

Add meat and remaining ingredients into the large bowl and toss well. Select Bake mode. Set time to 25 minutes and temperature 390 F then press START. The air fryer display will prompt you to ADD FOOD once the temperature is reached then place beef and broccoli in the air fryer basket. Serve and enjoy.

Spiced Pork Tenderloin

Preparation Time: 10 minutes Cooking Time: 35 minutes Serve: 6

Ingredients:

- 2 lbs pork tenderloin

For the spice mix:

- 1/2 tsp allspice
- 1 tsp cinnamon
- 1 tsp cumin
- 1 tsp coriander
- 1/4 tsp cayenne
- 1 tsp oregano
- 1/4 tsp cloves

Directions:

In a small bowl, mix together all spice ingredients and set aside. Using a sharp knife make slits on pork tenderloin and insert chopped garlic into each slit. Rub spice mixture over pork tenderloin. Sprinkle with pepper and salt. Select Bake mode. Set time to 35 minutes and temperature 375 F then press START. The air fryer display will prompt you to ADD FOOD once the temperature is reached then place pork tenderloin in the air fryer basket. Serve and enjoy.

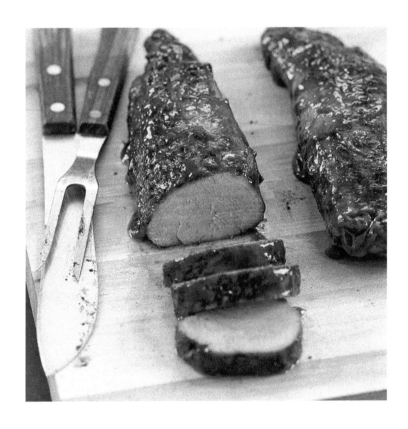

Spicy Pork Chops

Preparation Time: 10 minutes Cooking Time: 10 minutes Serve: 4

Ingredients:

- 4 pork chops
- 1/2 tsp black pepper
- 1/2 tsp ground cumin
- 1 1/2 tsp olive oil
- 1/2 tsp dried sage
- 1 tsp cayenne pepper
- 1 tsp paprika
- 1/2 tsp garlic salt

Directions:

In a small bowl, mix together paprika, garlic salt, sage, pepper, cayenne pepper, and cumin. Rub pork chops with spice mixture. Spray pork chops with cooking spray. Select Bake mode. Set time to 10 minutes and temperature 400 F then press START. The air fryer display will prompt you to ADD FOOD once the temperature is reached then place pork chops in the air fryer basket. Turn pork chops halfway through. Serve and enjoy.

Lemon Herb Lamb Chops

Preparation Time: 10 minutes Cooking Time: 16 minutes Serve: 4

Ingredients:

- 1 lb lamb chops
- 1 tsp coriander
- 1 tsp oregano
- 1 tsp thyme
- 1 tsp rosemary
- 2 tbsp fresh lemon juice
- 2 tbsp olive oil
- 1 tsp salt

Directions:

Add all ingredients except lamb chops into the zip-lock bag. Add lamb chops to the bag. Seal bag and place in the refrigerator overnight. Select Air Fry mode. Set time to 16 minutes and temperature 390 F then press START. The air fryer display will prompt you to ADD FOOD once the temperature is reached then place lamb chops in the air fryer basket. Turn lamb chops halfway through. Serve and enjoy.

Cajun Herb Pork Chops

Preparation Time: 10 minutes Cooking Time: 9 minutes Serve: 2

Ingredients:

- 2 pork chops, boneless
- 1 tsp herb de Provence
- 1 tsp paprika
- 1/2 tsp Cajun seasoning
- 3 tbsp parmesan cheese, grated
- 1/3 cup almond flour

Directions:

Mix together almond flour, Cajun seasoning, herb de Provence, paprika, and parmesan cheese. Spray both the pork chops with cooking spray. Coat both the pork chops with almond flour mixture. Select Bake mode. Set time to 8 minutes and temperature 350 F then press START. The air fryer display will prompt you to ADD FOOD once the temperature is reached then place pork chops in the air fryer basket. Turn pork chops halfway through. Serve and enjoy.

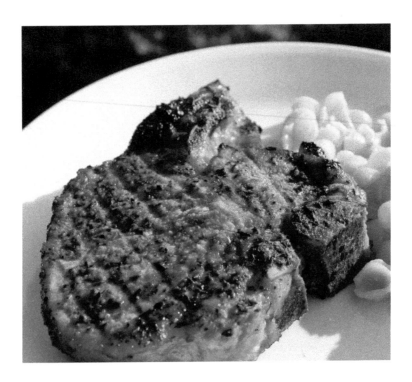

Thai Pork Chops

Preparation Time: 10 minutes Cooking Time: 12 minutes Serve: 2

Ingredients:

- 2 pork chops
- 1 tsp black pepper
- 3 tbsp lemongrass, chopped
- 1 tbsp shallot, chopped
- 1 tbsp garlic, chopped
- 1 tsp liquid stevia
- 1 tbsp sesame oil
- 1 tbsp fish sauce
- 1 tsp soy sauce

Directions:

Add pork chops in a mixing bowl. Pour remaining ingredients over the pork chops and mix well. Place in refrigerator for 2 hours. Select Air Fry mode. Set time to 12 minutes and temperature 400 F then press START. The air fryer display will prompt you to ADD FOOD once the temperature is reached then place marinated pork chops in the air fryer basket. Serve and enjoy.

Savory Dash Seasoned Pork Chops

Preparation Time: 10 minutes Cooking Time: 20 minutes Serve: 4

Ingredients:

- 4 pork chops, boneless
- 2 tbsp dash seasoning

Directions:

Coat pork chops with seasoning. Select Air Fry mode. Set time to 20 minutes and temperature 360 F then press START. The air fryer display will prompt you to ADD FOOD once the temperature is reached then place pork chops in the air fryer basket. Turn pork chops halfway through. Serve and enjoy.

Spicy Asian Lamb

Preparation Time: 10 minutes Cooking Time: 10 minutes Serve: 4

Ingredients:

- 1 lb lamb, cut into 2-inch pieces
- 1 tbsp soy sauce
- 2 tbsp vegetable oil
- 1/2 tsp cayenne
- 1 1/2 tbsp ground cumin
- 1/4 tsp liquid stevia
- 2 red chili peppers, chopped
- 1 tbsp garlic, minced
- 1 tsp salt

Directions:

Mix together cumin and cayenne in a small bowl. Rub meat with cumin mixture and place in a large bowl. Add oil, soy sauce, garlic, chili peppers, stevia, and salt over the meat. Mix well and place in the refrigerator overnight. Select Air Fry mode. Set time to 10 minutes and temperature 360 F then press START. The air fryer display will prompt you to ADD FOOD once the temperature is reached then place marinated meat in the air fryer basket. Serve and enjoy.

Chipotle Steak

Preparation Time: 10 minutes Cooking Time: 10 minutes Serve: 3

Ingredients:

- 1 lb ribeye steak
- 1/4 tsp onion powder
- 1/4 tsp garlic powder
- 1/4 tsp chili powder
- 1/2 tsp black pepper
- 1/2 tsp coffee powder
- 1/8 tsp cocoa powder
- 1/8 tsp coriander powder
- 1/4 tsp chipotle powder
- 1/4 tsp paprika
- 1 1/2 tsp sea salt

Directions:

In a small bowl, mix together all ingredients except steak. Rub spice mixture all over the steak and let sit the steak for 30 minutes. Select Air Fry mode. Set time to 10 minutes and temperature 390 F then press START. The air fryer display will prompt you to ADD FOOD once the temperature is reached then place steak in the air fryer basket. Turn steak halfway through. Serve and enjoy.

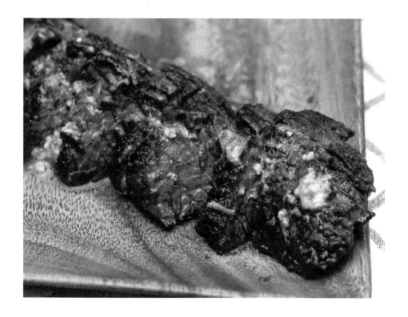

Baked Lamb Chops

Preparation Time: 10 minutes Cooking Time: 20 minutes Serve: 5

Ingredients:

- 5 lamb rib chops
- 1 garlic clove, grated
- 2 tbsp olive oil
- 1 tsp paprika
- 1/2 tsp smoked paprika
- 1 tsp cumin
- 1/2 tbsp oregano

Directions:

In a small bowl, mix together paprika, smoked paprika, cumin, oregano, garlic, and 1 tbsp olive oil. Coat lamb chops with spice mixture and place in the refrigerator for 3 hours. Heat remaining 1 tbsp olive oil in a pan over medium-high heat. Once the oil is hot then place lamb chops and cook for 3 minutes or until browned. Select Bake mode. Set time to 16 minutes and temperature 375 F then press START. The air fryer display will prompt you to ADD FOOD once the temperature is reached then place lamb chops in the air fryer basket. Turn lamb chops halfway through. Serve and enjoy.

Lemon Garlic Sirloin Steak

Preparation Time: 10 minutes Cooking Time: 30 minutes Serve: 6

Ingredients:

- 2 lbs sirloin steak, cut into
- 1-inch pieces
- 2 garlic cloves, minced
- 1 1/2 cups fresh parsley, chopped
- 1/2 tsp black pepper
- 3 tbsp fresh lemon juice
- 1 tsp dried oregano
- 1/4 cup water
- 1/4 cup olive oil
- 1 tsp salt

Directions:

Add all ingredients except beef into the large bowl and mix well together. Pour bowl mixture into the large zip-lock bag. Add beef into the bag and shake well and refrigerate for 1 hour. Select Bake mode. Set time to 30 minutes and temperature 400 F then press START. The air fryer display will prompt you to ADD FOOD once the temperature is reached then place marinated beef in the air fryer basket. Serve and enjoy.

Flavorful Air Fryer Kabab

Preparation Time: 10 minutes Cooking Time: 10 minutes Serve: 4

Ingredients:

- 1/2 lb ground beef
- 1/2 lb ground pork
- 4 garlic cloves, minced
- 1/2 tsp onion powder
- 1 tsp chili powder
- 1/4 tsp paprika
- 1/4 cup fresh parsley, chopped
- 1 tbsp olive oil
- 1 tsp salt

Directions:

Add all ingredients into the mixing bowl and mix until well combined. Place in refrigerator for 30 minutes. Divide mixture into the 4 portions and make sausage shape kabab. Select Air Fry mode. Set time to 10 minutes and temperature 375 F then press START. The air fryer display will prompt you to ADD FOOD once the temperature is reached then place kabab in the air fryer basket. Turn kabab halfway through. Serve and enjoy

Baked Lamb Patties

Preparation Time: 10 minutes Cooking Time: 15 minutes Serve: 4

Ingredients:

- 1 lb ground lamb
- 1 tsp chili pepper
- ½ tsp ground allspice
- 1 tsp ground cumin
- 1/4 cup fresh parsley, chopped
- 1/4 cup onion, minced
- 1 tbsp ginger garlic paste
- 1/4 tsp pepper
- 1 tsp kosher salt

Directions:

Add all ingredients into the large bowl and mix until well combined. Make four equal shapes of patties from meat mixture. Select Bake mode. Set time to 15 minutes and temperature 400 F then press START. The air fryer display will prompt you to ADD FOOD once the temperature is reached then place patties in the air fryer basket. Turn patties after 8 minutes. Serve and enjoy.

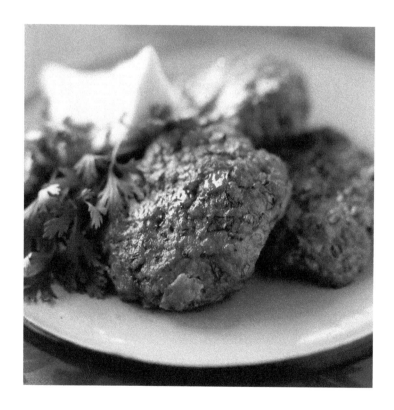

Greek Beef Casserole

Preparation Time: 10 minutes Cooking Time: 1 hour 30 minutes Serve: 6

Ingredients:

- 1 lb lean stew beef, cut into chunks
- 4 oz black olives, sliced
- 7 oz can tomatoes, chopped
- 1 tbsp tomato puree
- 2 cups beef stock
- 2 tbsp olive oil
- 1/4 tsp garlic powder
- 2 tsp herb de Provence
- 3 tsp paprika

Directions:

Heat oil in a pan over medium heat. Add meat to the pan and cook until browned. Add stock, olives, tomatoes, tomato puree, garlic powder, herb de Provence, and paprika. Stir well and bring to boil. Transfer meat mixture into the baking dish. Cover dish with foil. Select Bake mode. Set time to 60 minutes and temperature 350 F then press START. The air fryer display will prompt you to ADD FOOD once the temperature is reached then place the baking dish in the air fryer basket. Stir well and cook for 30 minutes more. Serve and enjoy.

Mini Meatloaf

Preparation Time: 10 minutes Cooking Time: 25 minutes Serve: 2

Ingredients:

- 1/2 lb ground beef
- 1 1/2 tbsp almond flour
- 1 egg, lightly beaten
- 2 olives, chopped
- 1 tbsp green onion, chopped
- 1/2 small onion, chopped
- 1 tbsp chorizo, chopped
- Pepper Salt

Directions:

In a large bowl, mix together all ingredients until well combined. Transfer meat mixture into the small baking dish. Cover dish with foil. Select Bake mode. Set time to 25 minutes and temperature 400 F then press START. The air fryer display will prompt you to ADD FOOD once the temperature is reached then place the baking dish in the air fryer basket. Serve and enjoy.

Flavorful Beef Satay

Preparation Time: 10 minutes Cooking Time: 8 minutes Serve: 2

Ingredients:

- 1 lb beef flank steak, sliced into long strips
- 1 tbsp fish sauce
- 2 tbsp olive oil
- 1 tsp hot sauce
- 1 tbsp Swerve
- 1 tbsp ginger garlic paste
- 1 tbsp soy sauce
- 1/2 cup parsley, chopped
- 1 tsp ground coriander

Directions:

Add all ingredients into the zip-lock bag and shake well. Place into the refrigerator for 1 hour. Select Air Fry mode. Set time to 8 minutes and temperature 400 F then press START. The air fryer display will prompt you to ADD FOOD once the temperature is reached then place marinated meat in the air fryer basket. Stir halfway through. Serve and enjoy.

Steak Fajitas

Preparation Time: 10 minutes Cooking Time: 15 minutes Serve: 6

Ingredients:

- 1 lb steak, sliced
- 1/2 cup onion, sliced
- 1 red bell peppers, sliced
- 1 yellow bell peppers, sliced
- 1 green bell peppers, sliced
- 1 tbsp olive oil
- 1/4 tsp chili powder
- 1 tbsp fajita seasoning

Directions:

Add all ingredients large bowl and toss until well coated. Select Air Fry mode. Set time to 15 minutes and temperature 390 F then press START. The air fryer display will prompt you to ADD FOOD once the temperature is reached then place fajita mixture in the air fryer basket. Stir after 10 minutes. Serve and enjoy.

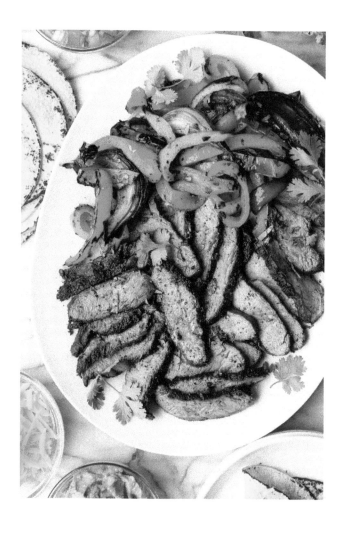

Buttery Steak Bites

Preparation Time: 10 minutes Cooking Time: 7 minutes Serve: 4

Ingredients:

- 1 lb steak, cut into
- 1-inch cubes
- 2 tbsp steak seasoning
- 4 tbsp butter, melted
- Pepper Salt

Directions:

Add steak, butter, seasoning, pepper, and salt into the bowl and mix well. Select Air Fry mode. Set time to 7 minutes and temperature 350 F then press START. The air fryer display will prompt you to ADD FOOD once the temperature is reached then add steak bites in the air fryer basket. Stir after 5 minutes. Serve and enjoy.

Greek Meatballs

Preparation Time: 10 minutes Cooking Time: 20 minutes Serve: 6

Ingredients:

- 2 lbs ground pork
- 1 egg, lightly beaten
- 1 tbsp lemon zest
- 1/4 cup shallot, diced
- 1 tsp garlic powder
- 1 tsp dried oregano
- 1 tsp dried thyme
- 1/4 cup bell pepper, diced
- 1/4 cup yogurt
- 1 cup feta cheese, crumbled
- 1 cup spinach, cooked, squeezed & chopped
- Pepper Salt

Directions:

Add all ingredients into the mixing bowl and mix until well combined. Make small balls from the meat mixture. Select Bake mode. Set time to 30 minutes and temperature 375 F then press START. The air fryer display will prompt you to ADD FOOD once the temperature is reached then place meatballs in the air fryer basket. Stir halfway through. Serve and enjoy.

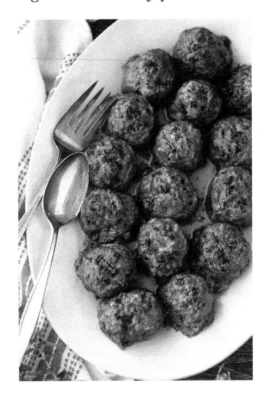

Pecan Crusted Pork Chops

Preparation Time: 10 minutes Cooking Time: 20 minutes Serve: 6

Ingredients:

- 1 1/2 lbs pork chops, boneless
- 2 eggs, lightly beaten
- 2 cups pecans, crushed
- 1/4 cup Dijon mustard

Directions:

Rub pork chops with mustard and set aside for 5 minutes. In a shallow bowl, whisk eggs. In a separate shallow dish, add finely crushed pecans. Dip pork chops in egg and coat with crushed pecans. Select Bake mode. Set time to 20 minutes and temperature 350 F then press START. The air fryer display will prompt you to ADD FOOD once the temperature is reached then place pork chops in the air fryer basket. Serve and enjoy.

Asian Pork Steak

Preparation Time: 10 minutes Cooking Time: 15 minutes Serve: 4

Ingredients:

- 1 lb pork steaks, boneless
- 1 tsp garam masala
- 1 tbsp ginger garlic paste
- 1/2 tsp cayenne
- 1/2 tsp ground cardamom
- 1 tsp cinnamon
- 1/2 onion, diced
- 1 tsp salt

Directions:

Add all ingredients except meat into the mixing bowl and mix well. Add the meat into the bowl and coat well. Place meat into the refrigerator overnight. Select Air Fry mode. Set time to 15 minutes and temperature 330 F then press START. The air fryer display will prompt you to ADD FOOD once the temperature is reached then place steaks in the air fryer basket. Turn halfway through. Serve and enjoy.

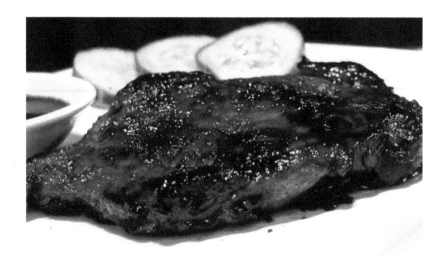

THANK YOU

Thank you for choosing *Low Fat Air Fryer Meat Meal Prep* for improving your cooking skills! I hope you enjoyed making the recipes as much as tasting them! If you're interested in learning new recipes and new meals to cook, go and check out the other books of the series.

CPSIA information can be obtained
at www.ICGtesting.com
Printed in the USA
BVHW091316010621
608554BV00008B/1134